Milk. Toast.

My Journey Managing Celiac Disease and Food Allergies at Home and on the Road

Heidi L. Smith
Certified Integrative Nutrition Health Coach,
Certified Meeting Professional

Milk. Toast.
My Journey Managing Celiac Disease and Food Allergies at Home and on the Road

To contact the publisher, visit
www.createspace.com

To contact the author, visit
www.integrativewellnessstudio.net

ISBN# **978-1523271436**
ISBN 10: 1523271434
Library of Congress Control Number: **2016903569**
Create Space Independent Publishing Platform, North Charleston, SC

Printed in the United States of America

This book is dedicated to those who have been diagnosed with food allergies and who struggle trying to manage their meals with family, friends, and colleagues. It is also for those who entertain a lot or travel and have had a hard time finding good things to eat that won't make them sick. This book will give you some tools and resources to create a healthy lifestyle that you can manage anywhere!

Contents

Acknowledgments

There are so many to thank for the opportunity to bring this book to life. First, to my amazing husband, Dennis, thank you for giving me the support and freedom to do this and for believing in me always. To my mother, Anke, for encouraging me to follow my dream and take a chance on doing something positive with something that was, at one time, such a negative in my life. To Bob and Paul for literally saving my life. If it were not for you both, I might not be here to share my story and to help others manage their life with celiac disease and food allergies, and I might not be here today enjoying the magic that is my life. I love you all!

Introduction

Having lived for years with undiagnosed autoimmune diseases that caused allergic reactions to both gluten and dairy (milk and toast), I suffered for many years and didn't know why. After finally being diagnosed with celiac disease and a serious dairy allergy but traveling constantly, I had to learn to manage my conditions when I was away from home, and that was not always easy.

The good news was that my diseases did not need surgery or medication. All I had to do was stop eating things that made me sick. Sounds easy enough, right? Not always. This book with give you some real tips and tricks to manage not only gluten and dairy allergies but others as well, while you are at home and on the road. It is a broader overview on how to eat healthier foods that will make your body feel great!

As Hippocrates said more than two thousand years ago, "[l]et food be thy medicine and medicine be thy food." Let's take a journey together to learn to manage your life without "milk and toast" and those food items that have been making you sick.

Chapter 1: My Story

My story started as that of a "gassy" child. Back then, my mother said I just had a sensitive stomach, and that was always, pretty much, end of conversation. My family was kind of flatulent, and we thought it was funny. Little did I know that it was a glimpse into my future with celiac disease and eosinophilic esophagitis (big words that we will get into later). It was not my mother's fault that I was gassy, but people just did not talk much about stomach issues in children back then—not that I can recall.

Through the years, my stomach troubles continued and seemed to worsen. I grew up on pasta, bread, pizza, milk, and meat—staples for the typical Midwestern family. It never occurred to me that these normal foods were making me sick or that they would have harmful long-term effects on my body, but it was happening right before my eyes.

I recall times when I would eat dinner and, almost immediately after the meal, I would be so bloated and uncomfortable that I looked like I was six months pregnant, and all I wanted to do was go poop! I know, that is a bit gross, but it is the truth.

When you are in your teens or early twenties, you can imagine how embarrassing and devastating it can be to feel like that after almost every meal! It never occurred to me to track what I was eating. It just seemed that it was my lot in life and that I had to deal with it.

As my career began in the meetings and convention industry and I began to travel a lot, I knew that I had to get a handle on what was going on when I ate. There was no way I could be on the road as often as I was, eating out and entertaining customers and feeling miserable each time I had a meal. My very first trip to the doctor was for a colonoscopy, prescribed by my doctor after several medications did not work. I was told that my condition was irritable bowel syndrome, or IBS. Quickly, the doctor gave me a prescription and told me not to drink so much coffee, and I was on my way.

Guess what? Nothing got better. And so it goes…

As time went on, I started to notice other things going awry in my body. In addition to the bloating and gas, now I was also noticing a really odd rash on my chin. I've never had acne a day in my life (good skin genes, I guess), but suddenly I noticed these small blister-like rashes on my chin. Of course, the normal thing to do is to run out for better skin-care products.

Guess what? Those did not work either.

Several years had passed, and I found myself not only traveling like a nut but also running my own business. I had amazing clients that had business for me all around the city and country. It was great! I traveled all the time and was entertaining nearly five days a week. Of course, I was eating all the wrong foods, drinking too much wine, and working about ninety hours a week. It was no surprise that at a certain point, I ended up very sick. Thinking it was stomach flu, I powered though it and kept working. My neighbors saw me one evening and commented that I looked pretty bad. "Thanks a lot," I thought. They asked how much weight I had lost. It really had not occurred to me that I had lost much weight, and I was kind of excited about the notion; in my head, a girl could always stand to lose another five pounds!

Immediately, I got on the scale and was horrified to see that I had lost sixteen pounds--in two weeks! Something was very wrong. In addition to my crazy work schedule, I was training for a run and had been carb loading. Oatmeal and fruit for breakfast, a veggie sandwich for lunch, and pasta with veggies for dinner. It seemed pretty healthy to me.

A few days later, I was supposed to be working a huge tradeshow for a client of mine but felt so weird in the morning that I went to see my neighbors again. One was a nurse, and the other a cardiology fellow. They suspected that I was very dehydrated and suggested that I head to the emergency room in the morning after a big bottle of Gatorade and a banana. So, first thing in the morning, with zero energy and tingling and numbness in my hands and face, I went straight to the ER. Yep, I was badly dehydrated and immediately hooked up to about four IV bags of fluids. I stayed home from the show for two days but felt very guilty about leaving my client to manage without me.

The last day of the show was upon me, and I managed to get up and shower, but when I tried to blow-dry my hair, I did not even have the energy to hold up the dryer. I leaned over the sink to hold my arm up and got the job done. What scared me was that when I went to put the dryer down, my hand wouldn't open! How weird is that? I was truly not thinking clearly at this point. I pried my hand open; thought, "I must need food and something to drink"; proceeded to fix a bagel and coffee for my trip to the show; and got behind the wheel of a car. Not too smart.

I arrived at the convention center, and as I walked into our show office, my client took one look at me and yelled to the team, "Call nine one one," Surely he was kidding. He was not. He told me that my lips were kind of blue, and he was not taking no for an answer. One of the team members had nursing training and took my vitals; it did not look good.

The EMTs arrived and swept me onto a stretcher. That was embarrassing because about five thousand people had begun to enter the tradeshow floor. The poor EMT tried for ten minutes to get an IV line into my arms, but my veins had collapsed from the dehydration, so I got a very painful needle in my foot, and I was about to spend some time in the hospital.

Arriving in the ER, I was greeted by an attending physician and about six medical students trying to surmise what my affliction was. All I recall was that the attending said if I had actually worked that day, I likely would have had dropped dead from a heart attack because my system had started to shut down from dehydration. My hand had not been working properly that morning because of it. Now it is all starting to make sense, but what was causing such bad dehydration?

After spending five days in the hospital, getting sicker and sicker, one gastroenterologist finally came to see me one evening with a large medical journal in hand. He showed me a list of symptoms and asked how many applied to me. I scored about a 98 percent, and he was certain that he knew what was wrong with me. Hallelujah! A simple blood test, and then I would have results in the morning.

I was so happy to see him that morning, so I could finally get out of the hospital. He had a diagnosis: celiac disease! "What in God's name is celiac disease?" I asked. He explained what it was, and I asked if I needed medication or surgery. His answer was simple. "Just stop eating things with gluten in them."

That was it? After all this and all these years, he simply said to stop eating foods with gluten.

That was the beginning of my journey with celiac disease.

What Is Celiac Disease?

Celiac disease is an autoimmune disorder that can occur in genetically predisposed people for whom ingesting foods containing gluten can lead to damage in the small intestine.

When people who have celiac disease eat gluten—a protein found in wheat, barley rye, and sometimes oats—their body has a serious immune response that essentially attacks the small intestine. The attacks damage the small, fingerlike projections in the intestine called villi. Villi are essential in promoting nutrient absorption, and when the villi are damaged, a person's body cannot properly absorb nutrients.

How Prevalent Is Celiac Disease?

Estimates show that worldwide, nearly one in one hundred people have celiac disease. It is estimated that nearly 2.5 million Americans go undiagnosed and are at risk for a variety of health complications.

According to the Celiac Disease Foundation, celiac disease is hereditary and runs in families. People with a first-degree relative with celiac disease (parent, child, sibling) have a one in ten risk of developing celiac disease. One in seven Americans may have some form of a gluten allergy or intolerance. The number of people in this country with either a sensitivity or full-blown celiac disease has grown exponentially since the 1950s. It is thought that the changes in how wheat is grown and processed have caused an increase in the prevalence of gluten issues. Changes in wheat grains and the way they have been processed and modified over the years help make the bread easier to slice, but the changes have been detrimental to a large group of Americans. We have sacrificed food quality for food convenience.

The tricky part about celiac disease is that it can manifest itself at any age. Any time a person starts eating foods or taking medicines that include gluten, it can prompt the beginning of noticeable symptoms. This disease cannot be left untreated because it may lead to other autoimmune disorders such as multiple sclerosis, type 1 diabetes, and anemia. It can also cause a skin rash that is sometimes itchy, referred to as dermatitis herpetiformis. It can affect bone health, can lead to osteoporosis, and can cause infertility and miscarriage. Neurological disorders such as epilepsy and migraines can occur along with intestinal cancers.

Other Long-Term Health Conditions

- Lactose intolerance and other dairy intolerances
- Vitamin and mineral deficiencies
- Central and peripheral nervous-system disorders
- Pancreatic insufficiency
- Intestinal lymphomas and other gastrointestinal (GI) cancers (malignancies)
- Gall-bladder malfunction
- Ataxia, epileptic seizures, dementia, neuropathy, myopathy, and leukoencephalopathy

Lots of big words to worry about, right? To add just a few more terms for you to remember, celiac disease is also known as celiac, celiac sprue, nontropical sprue, and gluten-sensitive enteropathy, according to the Celiac Disease Foundation.

If you suspect that you may have a gluten sensitivity or something more serious, a simple blood test can be done to measure the levels of antibodies that are associated with celiac disease, showing if a person has the condition. Occasionally the blood test may come back negative. If symptoms persist, it is important to continue investigating, and a doctor may recommend having an endoscopy or a colonoscopy done either to confirm the negative result or to confirm that there is, in fact, a hidden gluten sensitivity or celiac disease.

How Can You Treat It?

It would be great if you could treat celiac with medication, but you cannot, at least not yet. The only treatment for celiac is a strict commitment to adhere to a gluten-free diet. To avoid gluten, you must avoid foods with wheat, rye, and barley. For some, you also will have to avoid oats. Foods like bread, pasta, and beer will be no-no's. Some people have such severe conditions that even the smallest amounts of gluten, like crumbs from a toaster, can trigger a reaction and further damage their small intestines.

What Foods Have Gluten in Them?

As we mentioned previously, wheat is one of the main culprits in aggravating gluten issues. The Western diet is full of wheat products, but other forms of wheat can be enemies of the gluten sufferer:

• Wheat starch	• Einkorn
• Wheat bran	• Farina
• Wheat germ	• Emmer
• Couscous	• Farina
• Cracked wheat	• Fu (common in Asian foods)
• Durum	• Gliadin
• Graham flour	• Kamut
• Matzo	• Semolina
• Spelt	

OK, so after reading this list, you may be rolling your eyes and thinking, "What in the world can I actually eat now?" Don't fear. There is plenty you can still eat. I will help you create those good foods and incorporate them into your daily diet.

For example, if you are a pasta fan, look for buckwheat pasta. Buckwheat does not contain gluten, so as long as you prepare it with gluten-free sauces, and in a gluten-free environment, you can have pasta—and other dishes like buckwheat crepes, too.

So, the following are other culprits:

- Barley
- Bulgur
- Oats (oats themselves don't contain gluten, but they can be processed in plants that produce gluten-containing grains and so may be contaminated)
- Rye
- Seitan
- Triticale and mir (a cross between wheat and rye)
- Veggie burgers (you must look for those that specify that they are gluten-free)

You may be surprised to know that gluten can also be found in soy sauce, prepared chicken broth, malt vinegar, salad dressings, seasonings, spices, and prepared spice mixes. Gluten may also be found in products like lotions, shampoos, skin-care products, lipsticks, and vitamins. Once you are diagnosed with gluten sensitivity and/or celiac disease, you will want to become compulsive about reading labels. I read the label on everything I buy to make sure there is no hidden gluten. This task seems a bit daunting, but once you get used to doing it, it will become second nature.

Chapter 3: Dairy Allergy or Lactose Intolerant?

Another very common allergy is an allergy to cow's milk. It is most common in infants and young children and sometimes in adults as well. Lucky me, I am one of those adults with a dairy allergy as well as celiac disease, so you can imagine my displeasure when traveling and trying to manage both of those allergies when I am away from home.

According to Food Allergy Research & Education, or FARE, symptoms of a milk/dairy allergy can range from being mild like the hives to a severe reaction such as anaphylaxis. This potentially deadly disease affects as many as one in thirteen children in the United States, and approximately 2.5 percent of children under the age of three are allergic to milk. Most children who develop a milk allergy will do so before the age of one, and most children will actually outgrow their milk allergy as they age.

Some children have a higher level of cow's milk antibodies in their blood, and for these children, their milk allergy is likely to persist. A doctor can do a blood test to measure these antibody levels in a child who has a milk allergy to determine if he or she may outgrow the allergy.

What is the difference between a milk allergy and lactose intolerance? The difference is the immune system. For those people who have lactose intolerance, they are missing the enzyme lactase from their system. This enzyme breaks down the lactose in milk and dairy products. People with a lactose intolerance and not able to digest or breakdown dairy foods and can experience symptoms such as bloating, gas, cramps, diarrhea, and nausea. It is just plain uncomfortable, but it is not life threatening.

On the other hand, a milk or dairy allergy is more serious because it is an overreaction of the immune system to a specific food protein. When a person eats that food protein, it can trigger an allergic reaction that can range from being mild to very severe. Some symptoms of an allergy are rashes or hives, itching, swelling, trouble breathing, wheezing, or even a loss of consciousness. For some, it can even be fatal.

In my case, my allergic reaction to milk and dairy products triggers my immune system to respond with inflammation in my esophagus. The esophagus is the muscular tube that allows the food you to swallow to go from the mouth to the stomach. The reaction I have causes inflammation in my esophagus, which makes my esophagus swell, making it hard for me to swallow.

There is an actual name for this condition, eosinophilic esophagitis. In this inflammatory condition, the wall of the esophagus fills with large amounts of eosinophils, which are a type of white blood cell. These white blood cells are called leukocytes, and they are made in the bone marrow. These cells are just one of the types of cells that can cause inflammation.

Leukocytes are persistent little things, and they go kind of wild in the type of inflammation these allergic reactions cause. The white blood cells (leukocytes or eosinophils) become caught in tissues, such as the esophagus, the small intestine, or the stomach, when they are exposed to an allergen.

Some other things can cause the esophagus to inflame in this way. The most common is acid reflux. Acid reflux usually causes heartburn, but it can also cause a type of ulcer in the inner lining of the esophagus.

Other conditions may cause the symptoms of eosinophilic esophagitis, including viruses (herpes simplex); *Candida*, a type of fungi; and radiation therapy. Some medications that may get stuck in the esophagus, like tetracycline and antibiotics, may also cause the inflammation and irritation.

The concern is that one of the major symptoms of eosinophilic esophagitis is difficulty swallowing food. This is also called dysphagia. Essentially, food becomes stuck in the esophagus when it is swallowed. Other symptoms that people may experience include abdominal pain, coughing, vomiting, chest pain, or nausea.

To put it simply, allergens cause the eosinophils to increase, which causes the esophagus to swell. Food gets stuck, and it is uncomfortable and sometimes just plain painful to swallow. This kind of irritation can lead to scarring in the esophagus as well, which makes the condition more difficult to treat or alleviate.

It is important to know the difference and if you have a milk or dairy allergy, talking with your doctor about carrying an EpiPen (epinephrine auto-injector) to counter an anaphylaxis response is wise.

Food Allergy Research & Education (FARE) works on behalf of the 15 million Americans with food allergies, including all those at risk for life-threatening anaphylaxis. This potentially deadly disease affects one in thirteen children in the United States—or roughly two in every classroom. FARE is a 501(c)(3) nonprofit organization that was formed in 2012 as the result of a merger between the Food Allergy & Anaphylaxis Network and the Food Allergy Initiative.

Great news! Having a food allergy or a food restriction is not the end of the world. With the right information and the right tools, food that you thought you may never be able to have again doesn't have to be totally off limits! I'm not saying that eating things that make you sick is OK. What I am saying is that with a little bit of imagination and creativity, you can enjoy the same kinds of foods in a different way. You may even discover that the new foods you are eating are even better than what you were eating before.

The other thing you may discover is that you did not realize how badly you felt until you don't feel that way any longer. That was certainly my experience. Once I got used to my dietary restrictions, it became really fun to see what kind of substitutions I could make and how creative my menu planning could become.

One recommendation I would make, from personal experience, is to have your doctor do a full blood workup on you after your diagnosis. I found that I had been anemic for years before my diagnosis, and it was good to also learn about vitamin deficiencies in other areas. That way, I was able to focus on the very best foods I needed to incorporate into my new dietary lifestyle to make sure I had optimal nutrition.

With most new lifestyle changes, it is going to be important to have some goals and strategies in mind before you set out on this healthy new journey. Have a really clear plan in place will help to make a transition into a gluten-free, dairy-free, or anything-free lifestyle much less stressful and difficult. Your goal should be to create a sustainable plan for you and your family that you can manage on a daily basis and one that everyone can enjoy.

Sustainable Diet Checklist

Know why you are doing this! Know your reason for making these changes. Is it because you will damage your long-term health if you continue eating these foods? Is it because you feel that by eliminating certain foods you will lose weight? Is it because you are trying to manage the new dietary lifestyle to help someone else in your family?

Don't try to do it alone. It is important to make sure that those who are close to you are supportive of your new changes. The last thing you want is to have people close to you trying to sabotage your efforts. Explain to them why you need to make these changes, how they can be supportive, and what your plan is. Doing so will make it easy for everyone. Once they understand your true motivation and need to become healthy, they can become your biggest supporters. Also, look for a dietician or a certified health coach to help you

---

Gluten-Free Starter Foods

The foods listed here are gluten-free and are great basics to start your meal planning.

Stay focused on fresh, whole foods! Think about eating as many colorful foods as you can. Fruits and veggies are the foundation of *any* healthy and sustainable diet.

Fresh meats, poultry, fish

Eggs

Fruits

Vegetables

Rice

Potatoes

Milk and cheese

Beans, seeds and nuts in their natural form

manage your new plan. These professionals can offer you support, resources, and ongoing plans to make your transition easy, effective, and enjoyable.

Keep things simple. My advice is not to start out right away worrying about making all kinds of involved meals and trying to copy a favorite old recipe and try to substitute all kinds of other foods to recreate a favorite dish. Instead, start out slow and easy. There are some great "starter" foods (see insert below) that you can incorporate as your staple foods and then start to get more creative from there.

Research and learn. Start looking for resources on books, websites, and blogs that offer information and details on your particular dietary allergy/restriction. Social media has provided amazing access to a world of information. I have joined several Facebook groups, subscribed to specialty blogs, and found experts that can provide me information on YouTube and similar outlets. I've founds many wonderful books, podcasts, and lectures that have really given me great information and resources on how to better manage my particular conditions. It can also be a great way to connect with others experiencing the same thing you are, and you can develop a strong support network.

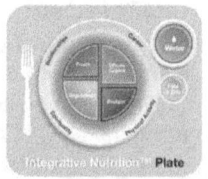

Don't freak out about mistakes! It happens, and it may happen a lot until you get used to your new lifestyle. All you can do is learn from the mistake, or the "miss"; make a plan so you know what to avoid next time; and move on.

If your condition is so severe that you will suffer an adverse reaction to even the slightest cross-contamination or contact, please make sure you know the ramifications and consult with your doctor/specialist to have a plan for getting you the care/treatment that you will need in an emergency.

Integrative Nutrition Food Plate

If you are at all like me, I find it helpful to have some guidelines regarding foods I should eat and how much on a daily basis. The Institute for Integrative Nutrition has a Nutrition Plate diagram that I find to make a lot of sense.

In this diagram, you will see that vegetables and whole grains are the largest portions and that proteins, followed by fruits, should be smaller portions. Instead of traditionally having milk or dairy as the accompanying beverage, this model prefers water as the beverage of choice. Most people do not drink enough water each day, and this is a great reminder to drink more water!

Fats and oils are not bad in this model either. The right portion of fats and oils are essential to a really healthy diet. Just don't overdo it and make sure that you are getting the right kind of fats and oils. I'll talk more about this later.

Use this plate as a reminder. It will help to keep you on track for eating a more balanced diet with the nutrients your body needs while avoiding the foods that you are not supposed to have.

Now we touched on the fact that fruits and veggies are naturally gluten-free so you can have as many of those as you wish. Remember to avoid any fruits and veggies that you are allergic to. I happen to have an unusual allergy to celery of all things, so I am sure to avoid that veggie. Not to mention the fact that I just plain hate the taste of it, I try very hard to make sure that I am not eating it in the foods that I am either making or selecting when I am out somewhere.

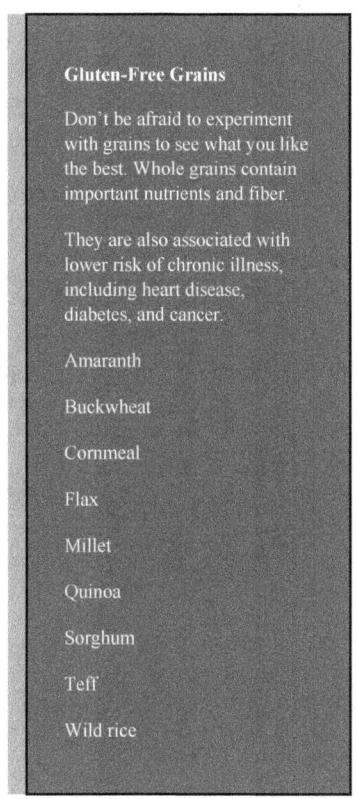

Gluten-Free Grains

Don't be afraid to experiment with grains to see what you like the best. Whole grains contain important nutrients and fiber.

They are also associated with lower risk of chronic illness, including heart disease, diabetes, and cancer.

Amaranth

Buckwheat

Cornmeal

Flax

Millet

Quinoa

Sorghum

Teff

Wild rice

Meats and other proteins are typically gluten-free in their natural state. Be careful, however, as there can be hidden gluten in certain protein foods. For example, some cold cuts and lunchmeats may contain wheat. Also beware that any breading, coating, or marinades may contain some gluten. I used to love using the imitation crab and lobster from the grocery for a quick salad until I discovered that those items also contain wheat. Read your labels! Look for hidden additives like wheat, gluten, soy, or monosodium glutamate when buying packaged meat, fish, and poultry.

Whole grain is the second-largest component to the Integrative Nutrition Food Plate. How do you manage to get the proper whole grain in your diet if you are allergic to gluten? This is where you need to be cautious about grains, but do not be discouraged. Foods made from wheat, barley, and rye all contain gluten. For some, oats pose a problem as well, so it is important to determine if oats are a problem for your system.

Many foods you probably know and love contain gluten. Bread, pasta, cakes, and cookies are just a few and probably the hardest ones for most with a gluten intolerance or celiac disease to give up. Here is the good news! Quite a few really good healthy grains are OK for you to eat.

Some of these grains may not be familiar to you, but most are prepared the same what that you would cook regular white rice. Consistency will vary on the type of grain, and you just need to experiment with the texture that you prefer.

Read Everything

The first step is to really understand if you or a loved one has an intolerance or an allergy. It will help to determine just how vigilant you need to be in making sure you are rid of your particular allergens in your home.

What you may not realize is that outside of the obvious food products like pasta, bread, and cookies, gluten may be lurking in some items that you may never expect. You will want to go through your pantry, your cupboards, and your bathroom closet searching for some hidden signs of gluten and, yes, I did say your bathroom closet.

It is likely that you will become the world's best label reader shortly after being diagnosed because you will need to look at every label to see if gluten may be among the ingredients. You can find it in baked goods, cereals, and frozen dinners. Those days of frozen Lean Cuisine or Swanson dinners are over because they all contain thickening agents in the sauces, which are off limits.

Gluten may also be found in soy sauce, gravy mixes, dry seasoning packets, salad dressing, pie filling, and other prepared foods. I thought I would cry when I found out that licorice contained gluten. I cannot tell you how long I had been eating red licorice whips when my world came crashing down! OK, that is a bit dramatic, but it was very upsetting because I am not a big candy eater but that was one of them.

Other Forms of Gluten/Wheat

- Dextrin
- Dinkle
- Durum
- Einkorn
- Emmer
- Farina
- Graham flour
- Kamut
- Semolina
- Spelt
- Wheat berry
- Wheat germ
- Wheat gluten
- Wheat bran
- Wheat starch

Some of the key words to look for include *wheat ingredient, wheat flour, wheat starch, barley extract, barley flavoring, malt, malt flavoring, malt extract, malt sugar, malt vinegar, rye, triticale,* and *wheat allergen.*

You will also want to look for products that contain gluten-free certification logos. Products marked with these logos have been tested for gluten, and ensures that it does not contain any gluten.

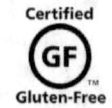

Each certification has its own symbol and requirements. There are several independent programs, such as those supported/backed by the Celiac Sprue Association, the Gluten-Free Certification Organization and the National Foundation for Celiac Awareness.

Be Aware of Cross-Contamination

Cross-contamination happens when gluten-free products are inadvertently mixed in with those containing gluten during milling, manufacturing, and/or shipping. If this happens, the gluten-free products become contaminated, and you need to be aware.

Some manufacturers will indicate the possibility of cross-contamination by having a disclaimer on the product that may say something like "produced in plant" that also processes wheat, soy, milk, nuts, or whatever the allergen is that you may be concerned about.

The US Food and Drug Administration (FDA) is working to make the format of these type of advisory labels more consistent so that it is easier for the consumer to find them on a product and to decipher what the danger of cross-contamination really may be.

Be aware that not everything is included in these cross-contamination warnings. Cross-contamination warnings are only obligated to the "Big 8" allergens, which are peanuts, tree nuts, milk, egg, wheat/gluten, soy, fish, and shellfish. It does not include things such as oats, rye, or barley, which also contain gluten, so be cautious.

You will now have to be your own detective and advocate. If you have products that are clearly marked and labeled gluten-free, you can feel confident that, according to the FDA guidelines, those products are safe to have in your home. If they do not, do your investigative work to determine if there is hidden gluten and/or any possible cross-contamination. If you are still unsure, contact the manufacturer. It is worth the extra effort to find out from the manufacturer directly if its product is safe as it will keep you and your family safe from any undo harm.

Find Other Resources

Some terrific shopping guides and mobile apps are available to help you to find safe products quickly and easily. Some that are easy to navigate and cost little to nothing include the following:

> Yummly Recipes and Grocery Shopping List
> Gluten-Free Shopping List
> Epicurious Recipes and Shopping List
> Celiac Shopping List and Gluten-Free Recipes
> Ceceliasmarketplace.com

The nice thing about these apps is that they are easy to take with you to the grocery store and it will help you to find specific brands that you can buy again and again. You will start to learn the manufacturers who cater to gluten-free or allergen-free products, and it will make your shopping easier. Be sure to update your apps updated regularly. Manufacturers will occasionally change their product ingredients and can do so at any time. You don't ever want to miss something has been added to one of your favorite products that is not good for you.

There are also some great websites for online shopping that you can use to buy small or large quantities of a wide variety of gluten-free products. The following are some such

> ww.udisglutenfree.com
>
> www.glutenfreemall.com
>
> www.eatgoodmarket.com

Medications/Vitamins/Dietary Supplements

Here is an area you may not have thought about initially regarding gluten. The sad fact is that gluten is hidden in many unlikely places, including medications, vitamins, and dairy supplements.

The adhesive supplements that bind together the contents of pills or tablets, called excipients, may contain gluten. An excipient is an inactive ingredient, which means that it has no medicinal effect, but it may contain dyes, preservatives, and flavoring agents. These additives may contain gluten so again, so be sure to read the labels on any of these type of products.

You will want to be sure and notify your pharmacists if you are taking any medications to see if those medications contain gluten. If so, you will need to see if there is an alternative option that is gluten free. Consult both your doctor and your pharmacist to work together on this for you.

The challenge with both prescription and over-the-counter medications is that they do not fall under the same gluten-free labeling rule. You can find any contaminants yourself by looking for some of the key ingredients such as the following:

- Wheat or wheat starch
- Modified starch (not specified as corn or any other gluten-free source)

- Pregelatinized starch (not specified as corn or any other gluten-free source)
- Pregelatinized modified starch (not specified as corn or any other gluten-free source)
- Maltodextrin (not specified as corn or any other gluten-free source)
- Dextri-maltose (may contain barley malt)
- Caramel coloring (may contain barley malt)
- Dextrin (typically comes from corn or potato but it is working looking into)

Vitamins and dietary supplements may be a bit easier to manage because they are regulated by the FDA and they also fall under and must comply with the Food Allergen Labeling and Consumer Protection Act (FALCAP). This act is the one that requires manufacturers to list common allergens (the Big 8) on their packages, including wheat/gluten. If a supplement is labeled as gluten-free, it must contain less than twenty parts per million of gluten. Again, check the label, and if you are still unsure, call the manufacturer directly.

Some of the vitamins that I really like that are gluten-free include the line of supplements from USANA. You can customize your vitamins and supplements based on your specific, bio-individual health needs. This company's processing methods and ingredients are really good, and it is the vitamin supplement brand that we prefer in my practice. Whatever brand you decide upon, just make sure that you have checked the ingredients and that they are safe for you and your family.

Be Diligent

It takes some time getting used to playing detective when it comes to the products your family now eats and uses on a daily basis. You will get the hang of it rather quickly, and it will become second nature once you know what to look for and where to look for it.

Where you will need to be a bit more concerned is when you buy food and products from places like your local farmers' market. If you are not sure if it contains gluten or your particular allergen of concern, ask! Local farmers' markets are now very often including suppliers who offer gluten-free and dairy-free foods. That so much more attention is being paid to these concerns is great because people who are managing food allergies can now participate in and enjoy local, fresh, and homemade offerings. Just be diligent about asking questions and investigating and then just enjoy!

Revamp Your Kitchen

Here is where the real work begins. It's time to revamp your kitchen. It is important, now that you know what to shop for, to set up your kitchen properly so that it is safe and free from gluten. When you first begin a gluten-free diet, focus on eating simple, healthy foods that are naturally gluten-free. The easiest way to do this is to cook at home more often. That way you know what you are cooking and what you are eating, and you can give yourself time to get used to your new way of eating.

Start with Foods Already in Your Kitchen

In general, this is a great exercise for making sure you are keeping items in your pantry and fridge on a rotation and not hoarding outdated and old products. Now you will want to take a little inventory of what is in your kitchen. Get out your guide of the key food items containing gluten and then begin going through your pantry, fridge, and freezer to eliminate those items with gluten. If you have any frozen entrees or frozen veggies with sauces, check those carefully as those typically contain gluten.

Look in the pantry for all the pasta, breads, crackers, cake/cookie mixes because they will have gluten in them as well. Be sure to look at cans of soups and any processed packaged food items like macaroni and cheese. This was a heartbreaker for me as it has gluten and dairy in it, but, thankfully, some gluten-free macaroni and cheese offerings are available that you and your kids will love!

Once you have all of the gluten tossed out of your kitchen by way of the packaged items, you will want to do a really thorough cleaning of the kitchen as well. Because all the food will be out of the cabinets and fridge anyway, this is a perfect time to go ahead and clean things out. Make sure to try to get rid all of the crumbs that may be lurking around and just thoroughly clean everything (I recommend using vinegar water as it is natural and free of chemicals) and then you have a clean kitchen to start cooking in.

Many of the foods that you already love are naturally gluten-free, so focusing on the things you already have and **can** have is great. Focus your shopping on things like fresh vegetables and fruits, rice, beans, lean meats, poultry, fish, milk, or substitutes such as soy, almond, rice, or cashew milk. Nuts, gluten-free condiments like mayonnaise, jellies/jams, and pickled and fermented foods are also great to have on hand. Be sure that these items are new and not already opened. If you have opened containers of things like mayonnaise, peanut butter, jelly, and other condiments that you would have used a knife or something to similar to get out of the container, toss it. These items may be contaminated with gluten, so it is better to be safe than sorry. Other items in this category that you will want to toss if opened are baking powder, sugar, and cornstarch. Don't forget to throw out any bags of flour that you have lying around because that is now a no-no.

If you want to keep the other food items containing gluten or your particular allergen, be sure to label them very clearly so that those with the allergy do not use them by mistake. As long as these items are not expired, you can give these them away to other family members or friends. For any unopened items, contact a local food pantry to see if it may be interested in taking the donation of unopened food products and pay it forward.

Clean It Up

Be sure to clean the kitchen well before you restock it will all of your healthy, new gluten-free items. Gluten can end up being a sticky and stubborn mess in your pantry and around the kitchen. Be sure to use a vacuum to get up all the crumbs hanging around in corners and crevices; clean out the refrigerator, stove, oven and microwave; wipe out all the cabinets and cupboards, including the drawer handles, and then buy new sponges, cleaning cloths and rubber gloves. All of your old ones may be contaminated with some gluten particles and, again, it is better to be safe than sorry.

Try not to be too overwhelmed with this whole process. It sounds like it is a lot of work and it can be. Break it up into stages, and then it seems easier to manage. One day, eliminate the gluten items from the kitchen. The next day, make it a cleanup day. On the third day, head to the grocery store and purchase the new food items you need. On the fourth day, cook your first simple-and-easy meal for your family! There will be recipes and other resources for you later in the book that you can try out in your newly appointed gluten-free kitchen.

Tools, appliances, and utensils can also cross-contaminate so you will want to pay attention to things like your toaster, cutting boards, wooden spoons, and strainers. If you will have some in your home who are gluten-free and some who will still consume gluten products, my suggestion would be to have a separate set of everything and label or use a different color for those items that are strictly gluten-free. Choose materials that are nonporous and easy to sanitize. Someone told me once to purchase red kitchen items for those that are gluten-free as it is an easy color to remember to "use with caution." Other kitchen items like bread makers, skillets, pancake griddles, and so on, can also harbor gluten and cross-contaminate. Pick everyday items like cutting boards to purchase right away and specialty items you use the most and replace those. Over time, you can keep on adding to your special gluten-free appliances until your kitchen wardrobe is complete.

Chapter 6: How Do I Manage My Food Allergies/Dietary Restrictions away from Home?

When I was first diagnosed with celiac disease, I worried about how I would manage my dietary restriction with my travel schedule for work. At the time, I was working in the meetings industry and was traveling a lot! When I say a lot, I mean that I was close to being one of those "road warrior" types who flew eighty thousand miles a year and knew the gate agents at O'Hare Airport by name. If I was on the road that much, how would I ever find anything I could eat that would not make me sick?

I must tell you, back then, it was difficult. At the time, early in the first decade of the twenty-first century, there weren't many products on the market, and there were certainly almost no restaurants serving gluten-free meals. Even more challenging was going to a conference, where the standard fare really consisted of bagels and Danish for breakfast, lunch was something with pasta and sauce on it, and dinner was usually eaten at a reception with passed hors d'oeuvres, of which about 90 percent of those were fried or served on a toast point. I was truly out of luck on most occasions and was not sure what to do.

It soon became very clear that now that I had taken care of managing being gluten-free at home, I had to do the same thing when I was on the road. So much of our daily lives take place away from home. Whether you are at work, traveling for business or pleasure, at business meetings, at children's activities, or at family outings, you will now need to learn, like I did, how to work around your dietary restriction and continue to live your life! The good news is that today, so many new products are on the market, more restaurants are recognizing the need for gluten-free options every day, and choices offered for vegans, vegetarians, and other dietary preferences are on the rise. Choices are now plentiful!

Things to remember when you will be away from home are to plan ahead, ask a lot of questions, and be prepared. Ultimately, you are responsible for your own health and wellness when you are away from your home environment. You can do some things in advance to make sure that your experience is easy, safe and pleasurable.

The first thing I suggest is to go into things with a positive and proactive mind-set. A gluten-free or other "free" diet does not have to put a damper on your experience away from home. Keep in mind that you just don't have control over some things and some situations. For those you can control, don't be afraid to ask questions and look for alternatives. Be sure that no matter what situation you find yourself in, you need to be prepared with something you can eat that is safe for you.

Carry an Allergy Card with You

Allergy cards are a great resource to keep with you when you are traveling and dining out. You can hand them to your waitstaff and/or to the chef to explain exactly what your allergy is or allergies are if you have more than one. They can also be translated into different languages in the case that you are traveling internationally.

There is a variety of resources for the allergy cards, and my favorite one is SelectWisely.com. On this website, you can choose from a variety of allergies and restrictions that are available. For example, this site has cards for food, drug, and skin-contact allergies. It also has cards for vegetarian, vegan, and other special diets. Cards for diabetes and other health emergencies are also available, so it is a pretty robust resource.

Your allergy information can be translated into just about any language, and the company will print the card and ship it to you. Or you can choose the e-mail option, and the created card will be e-mailed to you. Then all you do is print it out and then have it laminated, which keeps the card intact longer.

Another good resource is a do-it-yourself option at www.foodallergy.org. There is a tab for Safe FARE: Chef Card Template. In this area, they have standard verbiage to alert staff of your allergy and of what can happen. You fill in the blank area with the items you are allergic to, and then you can print it and have it laminated. You can just do one and keep it with you, but be sure to ask for it back each time you use it. Or you can print several and hand them out. If someone keeps it, you will still have others available. It just depends on your budget and on how frequently you think you will use the card.

My husband and I are going on vacation this summer to Greece and Italy, and so I went to SelectWisely.com and printed one in English, Greek, and Italian. This way, I will be covered no matter where we are, and then a particular establishment can let me now if they are able to accommodate my request or not. I'll be traveling with gluten-free foods just in case establishments cannot make me a special meal so that I will be prepared either way.

How to Enjoy Dining Out

Restaurants, banquet halls, and other public venues are not always equipped to prepare safe gluten-free or allergy-free foods. Again, the first thing to do is call ahead. Ask if the venue is able to accommodate your particular needs before you go. That way, you will know what your options are ahead of time and you can be prepared.

Because being gluten-free has become such a trend recently, some people who request a gluten-free meal may only be doing so because it happens to be the latest "fad diet" they are following. This would be someone who has a gluten-free food preference. Some others may have a gluten intolerance and will request a gluten-free meal but may not have any kind of serious issue if the restaurant cross-contaminates the food with something that has gluten in it. For those who have a serious gluten allergy or something like celiac disease, they will need to sure there is no cross-contamination in the facility and that they foods have no trace of gluten in them or it could be life threatening. The same thing goes for other allergies, particularly to things like peanuts, shellfish, and dairy.

The only way that a kitchen in a restaurant or another public facility can produce truly gluten-free food is if they have a totally separate area to prepare gluten-free foods. The grill has to be separate, storage of foods needs to keep gluten away from any other types of food with gluten in them and all utensils and cookware must be completely separate from those used to prepare regular meals.

So many restaurants list their menus online now that you can use that as a starting point. Check to see if there are gluten-free items on the menu. If there are, call and ask if they have a separate gluten-free food prep area or a gluten-free kitchen. If they do not, you know you have a risk of cross-contamination. If they do not have any gluten-free options on the menu, you can still call to see if there is something the chef can prepare for you that is safe for you to eat.

If living gluten-free is new to you, or if you have a multitude of allergies, bring your dietary guidelines with you in case you need to double-check what you can and cannot have to eat. In time, this will all become second nature. You won't think twice about asking those questions, and you will learn what ingredients and foods to look for and avoid. In the meantime, here are some helpful questions you can ask when dining out:

- Do you have gluten-free options?
- If not, are there any dishes that can be prepared gluten-free?
- Do you have a separate gluten-free kitchen, and how to you prevent cross-contamination?
- What are the ingredients in this dish?
- Have any special seasonings been used? (Some spices contain gluten)
- Have any items been coated or dusted with flour?
- Are your fried foods done in a separate fryer from other foods?
- Do your salads include croutons, or is my meal served with bread? If so, ask the server to not include these items.
- How are things like vegetables or rice cooked? In broth, stock, or water? Some broths and stocks already prepared contain gluten.
- For breakfast, is any flour or wheat added to the egg mix in scrambled eggs or omelets?
- What ingredients are in the salad dressing? Does it contain dairy or gluten from things like wheat or barley?

Sometimes asking this many questions in person can make you feel uncomfortable, particularly if you are with a lot of people or at a business function. Doing this ahead of time and then being prepared will make the entire experience more pleasant for you and your server.

The Best Way to Order

If you have not called in advance and ordered a special meal ahead of time, don't be afraid to let your server know what your restrictions are and what you can and cannot eat. If you have a serious condition such as celiac, be sure to let your server know that you have a potentially dangerous reaction to anything with gluten in it.

Because celiac is really an autoimmune disease and not an allergy, the server may not know, and telling him or her that you have an autoimmune disease may not register as being a bad thing. In this case, you may want to tell your server that you are allergic to gluten or dairy or whatever your allergy is so that he or she is aware that by eating it, you may become ill. Restaurants do not want you to get a meal you cannot eat, and even more so, they do not want you to have a meal that will make you sick, so do not be afraid to talk with your server.

As a rule, try to avoid any foods that are battered, fried, or in a sauce or gravy. These items will most typically contain gluten, so it is easier just to stay away from them. Avoid pasta, breads, and anything breaded unless the items are specifically noted as being gluten-free.

Also check on things like soup bases and dressings because they are often made using gluten. The server can tell you or find out if they are. If so, ask for an alternate such as vinegar and oil or oil and lemon juice because some vinegar may also contain gluten. I have found that it is easy to carry a small container of homemade dressing along, depending on where I'll be dining. The other things I always carry with me are individual packets of gluten-free soy sauce. I love Asian foods and so the gluten-free soy (Tamari) comes in handy if I am grabbing a quick lunch and need to use some. You can find those in some local grocery store chains and you can also order them online through a variety of retailers.

One more thing you can do, in a pinch, if a venue does not seem to be very accommodating is to stick to plain foods: salads without crouton or dressing, plain vegetables, plain potatoes and a grilled or baked piece of meat or fish. You may get a server or a chef who rolls his or her eyes at you if you ask about leaving off the fabulous sauces, and so on, but you aren't worried about his or her health. Order what will keep you healthy and happy! Ultimately, they want you to be satisfied with your experience, and a good server will try to accommodate, especially when tips are involved.

Another strategy you can use before you head out for dinner is to take a look at some different apps that are available to help you decipher what foods are gluten- or allergy-free at certain restaurant chains.

One that I use on a regular basis is Is That Gluten Free? Eating Out. This app lists many menu items for some major restaurant chains times. It will tell you if the food item is gluten-free and if that is verified or unverified. One that I find helpful that you can use in general and not just for a specific restaurant is called iEatOut. When you set up your account, it allows you to plug in the different allergies you may have. Then the app will allow you to pull up a specific ethnic meal choice such as Chinese food. It will then list some of the most popular dishes in that category and will tell you if any of the foods you are allergic to are in a particular dish. Pretty cool!

For example, I want Chinese food and would like to have some egg-drop soup. When I pull up that menu item, it shows me that it contains gluten and wheat. Now I know that egg-drop soup is off limits for me. Another of my favorite dishes is lemon chicken. This app shows that this particular dish may contain gluten and wheat. If you click on it again, it gives a description of how the dish is likely to be prepared. Then it gives you a list of decision factors to think about and/or ask about prior to ordering the dish. Here are some of the factors they list:

- Ensure no soy sauce—order gluten-free soy sauce if available.
- Ensure chicken is not battered or dusted with wheat flour. Ask if cornstarch or a gluten-free flour can be used instead (rice flour would be good).
- Ensure that stocks and broths are not made from bouillon, which may contain gluten.
- Ensure that oil used for frying has not been used to fry other items that may have been battered or dusted with wheat flour.

If the restaurant can accommodate those needs, then order the lemon chicken. If they cannot, you should consider ordering another dish.

Eating at Business Functions or Other Catered Events

I may be starting to sound like a broken record, but in all honesty, communication is the key to just about everything when you have any special dietary request.

When I was traveling a lot for work, I would find myself going to conferences and meetings for days at a time. Conference planners always seemed to serve a continental breakfast (sometimes a sit-down meal), and then lunch, and most often a reception or an occasional plated dinner. Breakfast was typically bagels and Danish and maybe some yogurt (none of which I can eat). Lunch was always up for grabs and usually included pasta, breads, and sauces. Again, I couldn't eat anything unless I ordered a plate of roasted vegetables. The hardest was dealing with the receptions because the hors d'oeuvres are often passed around and consist of foods like a bruschetta, something made with cheese, and lots of fried foods because these are easy and cheap to prepare. Again, I was going hungry.

After putting myself through that and having to either go hungry or find somewhere else to eat during the conference, I started to ask the event organizer more questions ahead of time. Things I would ask are, "Will the meal be plated, or is it a buffet?" and "Will there be any gluten-free and dairy-free options available?" and "Is it possible to order a special meal that is gluten-free and dairy-free?" The event planner is usually happy to share that information with you and will let you know what the capabilities are available to accommodate your needs. If I knew there wouldn't be many options for me, I would either find something to eat prior to the event or bring a special protein shake and snacks with me that I knew I could have in a pinch if I needed them.

In general, fruits and vegetables are usually safe, as is the cheese tray (unless you have a dairy issue like I do). Simply prepared meats or fish, without sauces, are also usually OK. If you have a question about any item and don't know, just avoid it, and try to find something else.

What if Your Travels Are Overseas?

Same rules apply overseas as they do here in the United States. Communication! Do research ahead of time to determine which hotels, resorts, tour groups, cruise lines, and airlines will be able to address your dietary needs. Surprisingly, many countries in Europe and around the globe are better at accommodating certain allergies and restrictions than we are here in the United States. There are even specialty travel clubs such as gluten-free, kosher, and vegetarian travel clubs, to name a few.

Once you settle on a hotel or a place to stay, ask about local restaurants and grocery stores that may have products available for your specific needs. Again, pack a stash of snacks and foods that you know are safe to eat; put them in your travel bag and/or carry-on. That way, no matter where you are or what resources are available, you know that you have something to keep you from going hungry. Be sure to bring enough in case of travel delays, and make sure you are covered at least for the trip there and the trip back. In most cases, you will be able to find something while you are in your destination that will satisfy your needs.

If your allergy is severe enough to need medication, don't forget to pack that as well. Always have on hand a stash of antihistamines, skin rash medications, and, if needed, an EpiPen. You never want to be caught in a situation where you could not find the medication you may need to save your life.

A website that I found to have some helpful tips and information on it about traveling with allergies is www.independenttraveler.com. It offers some good suggestions for what to do and to prepare for when traveling internationally. Just be aware of foods that are not allowed to be brought across borders so you don't run into an issue at the airport.

The following some of my favorite foods to take on trips:

- Dried fruits
- Homemade trail mix
- Gluten-free rice crackers
- Gluten-free protein or energy bars like Kind bars
- Snack bags of unsalted almonds for energy (plain are best as the salt can make you puffy on a flight)
- Allergy-free protein-shake packs like Arbonne Protein Mix (these are great as you just add to cold water and shake it in a shaker cup—always one in my suitcase)

As I mentioned earlier in Chapter 6, bring along an allergy card that has been translated into the language of the country you will be visiting. It will help the locals to understand better exactly what your needs will be during your stay.

Chapter 7: What Should I Do if I Am Entertaining?

If you are anything like me, you may find this part of being gluten-free or having dietary restrictions to be the most challenging. Unless you have several friends or family members who also have dietary restrictions, you will now become the one person they all will worry about feeding at gatherings. I've had celiac for more than fifteen years and my family still does not quite get it. It has gotten to the point that, depending where I am going, I often offer to bring a few dishes and usually bring some kind of gluten-free crackers or things like that for snacking.

Talk to whoever is hosting the event in advance to see what he or she plans to serve. If the host is serving pasta, for example, ask if he or she could use gluten-free pasta instead and then recommend the pasta brand that you like so the host has a level of confidence in what he or she would buy for you at the grocery store.

The other option is to explain what your particular condition can do to you if you eat it so they fully understand the seriousness of your request. Most of the time, they want you to be able to eat something and will work to accommodate your needs in some manner.

Remember to keep an eye out for cross-contamination and watch out for yourself. Example, if you are having breakfast together and they have a regular toaster for bread containing gluten, do not put your gluten-free bread into the same toaster or you risk cross-contamination. Let's say you have a dairy allergy and the family is serving ice cream for dessert, be sure to bring your own dairy-free ice cream before you arrive and ask that you have that instead of the regular one. I have found that if I bring along my own foods or dishes to a family gathering, I am not asking the host to spend the extra time and money to find and purchase specialty foods that only I will need, and he or she is usually not be bothered by that at all.

When people come to my house, it is much easier because I am in charge of what is being served. Some people will not eat anything if they know it is either gluten-free or dairy-free because they assume it just won't taste good. So, very often, I will make dishes that accommodate my dietary lifestyle and will not tell my guests. They usually never know the difference!

Gluten-free and dairy-free foods have come so far over the years that the quality and taste are really quite good. I have had pastas and pizzas that are totally gluten-free, and if I hadn't known that it was a gluten-free product, I would not have known the difference.

When you are the host, be sure to know your guests and what food allergies or dietary restrictions may your guests be dealing with so you can take them into consideration when planning your meals. I usually ask that when invitations are sent out whether it is verbally, via e-mail or on a platform such as Evite. Guests will be thankful that you care enough to ask, and when it is your turn to be entertained at their home, they are far more likely to take your needs into account as well.

As a rule, I try to prepare something for everyone. Some dishes will be gluten-free, some dairy-free, and some will be regular old original recipes without concern for dietary issues. I also like to keep things light when possible, so I do very little frying and include very few sauces and gravy. There are occasions, however, that I will cook things that I am never supposed to eat. My husband begs me to do my famous garlic-and-blue-cheese mashed potatoes, and I agree to make them—at Christmas. He will usually only get them once a year. They are ridiculously good, and just because they are not good for me does not mean that I would keep them from my husband or family. I have been known to stick the spoon into the pot to taste them before serving, and that is usually enough for me to get the taste and flavor of such a rich and decadent side dish without making myself sick from my dairy allergy.

Again, when it comes right down to it, get-togethers are really about the company you are with and sharing time together, not the food you will be eating. Appreciate your host for being willing to accommodate your special needs and enjoy the time with friends and family. You can always eat before you go and when you get home if all else fails.

Let's go back to some things I covered in chapter 5 regarding what you should avoid with a diagnosis of celiac disease or a gluten allergy or sensitivity:

- Barley (malt, malt flavoring, malt vinegar)
- Rye
- Wheat
- Triticale (cross between wheat and rye)
- Oats *

Now I have starred (*)oats because many doctors recommend that you avoid oats as well because they may be contaminated during the growing and processing procedures.

Also be sure to avoid food additives like modified food starch and medications and vitamins that contain gluten.

Wheat products can be listed as other things so be on the lookout for the following:

- Durum flour
- Farina
- Graham flour
- Kamut
- Semolina
- Spelt

Studies show that one out of every one hundred people in North America is thought to have celiac disease, and according to Dr. Peter Green, director of the Celiac Disease Center at Columbia University, between 10 and 20 percent of those with the autoimmune disease also have some degree of lactose intolerance. Interesting, isn't it? This really makes it a double-whammy for the person having to manage a new dietary lifestyle.

Dr. David Clark, functional neurologist, recommends that anyone with an autoimmune condition must *not* eat what he calls the "Unholy Trinity":

- Gluten
- Dairy
- Soy

Here is why Dr. Clark recommends a dietary lifestyle free of gluten, dairy, and soy: "When you have a sensitivity to gluten or any of the wheat compounds, you begin making antibodies to them. An antibody, if you want to think about it this way, is like an adhesive flashing strobe light made to stick to a specific invader (gluten/wheat compounds in this example)."

"So, for example, as a child, if you had chicken pox, you were exposed to chicken pox, and your body made antibodies to the chicken pox that will only stick to the chicken pox; therefore, you have an immunity to it" said Dr. Clark.

If you have a gluten-sensitivity problem, when you eat gluten, your body makes these antibodies. The antibodies find the gluten, and they bind onto it. The antibodies flash and tell your T-cells, "Hey, come on in and destroy this invader that we found. That's essentially what happens when you have a problem with gluten. So what I'm telling you about applies to anyone that has any type of gluten problem."

There's a problem with milk products called cross-reaction. The antibodies that are for gluten—they're only supposed to stick to the gluten—can actually stick to things that are not gluten and cause your immune system to have the same type of gluten immune system response.

To your immune system, the "cross-reacting" food is the same thing as gluten. So you could be on a gluten-free diet *but* also be consuming milk, which is a known cross-reactor. The milk fat and the milk proteins are close enough to gluten for your immune system to "cross-react" and close enough for gluten antibodies to bind onto and direct your immune system to try to kill this non-gluten food.

The result? You suffer an inflammatory reaction as if you were still eating gluten.

In my practice, I've seen a lot of people who had been doing well on a gluten-free diet but have kind of plateaued. Most of these people, when I finally got them to go on a milk product-free diet, they felt 30 to 40 percent better.

I am a perfect study on this theory. I had been lactose intolerant since back in college but did not really start paying attention to it until I was in my early twenties. When lactose-free milk finally came out, I was all over it and drank it every day. My symptoms never seemed to get better. Once I was diagnosed with celiac and began to do some research, I read that there is sometimes a correlation between those with celiac and a dairy allergy.

Several years ago, I was having some issue swallowing and noticed that when I would eat and sometimes even when I was drinking water, I felt as if it was getting stuck in my throat, and it was very hard to swallow. Trying not to panic about being diagnosed with yet another issue, I went to my gastroenterologist to have him see what was going on. It turned out that what I had thought was just a lactose intolerance was a full-blown dairy allergy. That dairy allergy was causing the white blood cells in my esophagus to become irritated and inflamed, hence, my difficulty in swallowing. That new development was called eosinophilic esophagitis (EoE). Delightful! One more condition I was going to have to deal with.

The main symptoms of this condition actually mimic GERD (gastroesophageal reflux disease). You may have heard of that condition because there are few over-the-counter medications for treating GERD, and they are not effective on EoE. Symptoms may include things like a general cough or pain in the chest, throat, or abdomen. Other symptoms include gas, bloating, and/or diarrhea and lower gastrointestinal symptoms.

I used to think that I just ate too fast or did not chew my food properly, and that was why I was feeling such a strange "choking" in my esophagus. It turned out that it was all tied in with my celiac disease and my dairy allergy. After struggling with it for many years and ignoring it, I finally had an upper endoscopy and an esophageal biopsy done, which confirmed my diagnosis.

There are several treatments for EoE, including a few dietary plans along with medical treatments such as using swallowed inhaled steroids. One of the treatments for EoE is what is called the Six Food Elimination Diet. Essentially, this diet requires eliminating six of the eight most common foods seen in allergic diseases. The specific foods are milk, egg, wheat soy, peanuts/tree nuts, and seafood (fish/shellfish). In my particular case, I was told to eliminate wheat/gluten, which I was already doing, and then to eliminate dairy altogether.

No medications are currently approved to treat EoE. However, some medications have been shown to reduce the number of eosinophils in the esophagus and improve symptoms. The most helpful medication in controlling inflammation in the esophagus is a glucocorticosteroid. The most common treatment is to swallow a corticosteroid instead of inhaling it. Depending on the severity of the inflammation, higher doses may be needed but that may also lead to a greater risk of side effects.

According to the American Academy of Allergy Asthma and Immunology, another course of detection and treatment may be the use of a proton-pump inhibitors. The proton-pump inhibitor essentially controls the amount of acid produced. Some patients respond well to the proton-pump inhibitors and can experience a significant decrease in the number of eosinophils and the amount of inflammation when also followed up with an endoscopy and biopsy. However, proton-pump inhibitors can help to improve EoE symptoms without making the inflammation any better. Researchers are now looking into using them to manage symptoms of EoE. Finding a doctor who specializes in conditions such as EoE and one who is knowledgeable in treating EoE is very important.

Now I do not claim to know enough to offer medical advice to anyone, but I do know that for me, the only way that I was going to see relief and to heal from my various conditions was to move to a dietary lifestyle that excluded gluten, dairy/casein, and as much sugar as possible.

There is a very strong tie between autoimmune disease and a leaky gut. The leaky gut, which I look at in the next chapter, can be healed by removing food triggers from one's diet. Those triggers include foods like sugar, dairy/casein, Genetically Modified Organisms, sugar, and un-sprouted grains. Are you beginning to see how all of these things are related?

For those who are trying to manage a gluten-free and dairy-free lifestyle, I highly recommend, as a rule, **eliminating all gluten, all dairy/casein, sugar, and adding in probiotic-rich foods.** When these food items are eliminated from your diet and, as long as you have no other allergies or health concerns, you can experience a dramatic change in your gut health and in the way you feel overall.

First, let's definite what Leaky Gut Syndrome is and then we will talk about how Leaky Gut ties into diseases like Celiac and other autoimmune diseases.

According to Dr. Andrew Weil, "Leaky Gut Syndrome is not generally recognized by conventional physicians, but evidence is accumulating that it is a real condition that affects the lining of the intestines. The theory is that leaky gut syndrome (also called increased intestinal permeability), is the result of damage to the intestinal lining, making it less able to protect the internal environment as well as to filter needed nutrients and other biological substances."

So, as a result, some bacteria, toxins, proteins not completely digested, fats, and waste not normally absorbed may "leak" out of the intestines into the bloodstream. This process triggers an autoimmune reaction, which can lead to gastrointestinal problems. Some common symptoms like abdominal bloating, excessive gas and cramps, fatigue, food sensitivities, joint pain, skin rashes, and autoimmunity may occur. The cause of this syndrome can be triggered by a variety of sources, such as chronic inflammation, food sensitivity, damage from taking large amounts of nonsteroidal anti-inflammatory drugs (NSAIDS), cytotoxic drugs, radiation, certain antibiotics, excessive alcohol consumption, or a compromised immunity.

In reality, we all have some degree of intestinal permeability. Based on what we eat, what our medical conditions are and what kind of lifestyle or bloodline we carry, we may be predisposed to a higher degree of permeability which leads to inflammation and can develop into conditions such as food sensitivities or allergies and/or autoimmune diseases.

Leaky gut has been found in association with asthma, diabetes, rheumatoid arthritis, irritable bowel (inflammatory bowel disease, or IBD, which includes Crohn's disease and ulcerative colitis), lupus, hypothyroidism, kidney disease, multiple sclerosis, psoriasis, eczema, depression, chronic fatigue syndrome, heart failure, and celiac disease. That is a large number of different diseases associated with a leaky gut!

Another thing that causes leaky gut syndrome is antibiotics. Not only are they overprescribed in this country, but they are also destroying our gut health. Antibiotics destroy beneficial bacteria living in our bowels by allowing bile salts to enter and damage the large intestine. This may be one of the reasons we are seeing higher incidences of colon cancer in our society.

Antibiotics also promote the growth of Candida and other fungi and yeast in the body. What is Candida? The *Merriam-Webster Dictionary* defines Candida as the following:

*any of a genus (*Candida*) of parasitic fungi that resemble yeasts, occur especially in the mouth, vagina, and intestinal tract where they are usually benign but can become pathogenic, and have been grouped with the imperfect fungi but are now often placed with the ascomycetes; especially: one (*C. albicans*) causing thrush.*

The real damage done by *Candida* is to the epithelial barrier of the intestine, which then allows the absorption of toxins and chemicals that then enter the blood and can affect a number of different organs in the body, including the brain.

Donna Gates, MEd, ABAAHP, is the international best-selling author of *The Body Ecology Diet: Recovering Your Health and Rebuilding Your Immunity*. Donna is on advanced fellow with the American Academy of Anti-Aging Medicine. She is on a mission to change the way the world eats. *The Body Ecology Diet* was the first book of its kind—sugar-free, gluten-free, casein-free, and probiotic rich. In 1994, Donna introduced the natural sweetener stevia to the United States, began teaching about fermented foods, and coined the phrase "inner ecosystem" to describe the network of microbes that maintains our basic physiological processes—from digestion to immunity. Over the past twenty-five years, Donna has become one of the most respected authorities in the field of digestive health, diet, and nutrition.

One of the dietary theories I have studied in my practice is one created by Donna Gates called the Body Ecology Diet. Now I am not here to necessarily recommend the products that she sells within her program but rather I am here to make you aware of the theory within that dietary lifestyle, which basically says that to overcome Candida and yeast within our bodies and to heal infection and disease it is imperative to eliminate gluten, dairy/casein, and sugar and to have a diet rich with probiotics to heal your gut health. This goes back to my recommendation chapter eight that states that following these guidelines will heal your gut and, subsequently, will begin to heal other conditions you may have been dealing with for a long time.

There are four easy steps you can take to begin healing your leaky gut and they are pretty intuitive.

Step 1: Remove trigger foods.

If you are allergic to any food, you will need to eliminate that food completely. If there are certain foods that irritate your gut but you may be not allergic by eliminating them, you will get closer to healing.

Step 2: Replace trigger foods with healing foods.

This list of healing foods will help to heal your leaky gut and will rebuild the health of your immune system.

Bone Broth: contains collagen and the amino acids proline and glycine that can help heal your damaged cell walls. I've had many of my patients do a bone broth fast for three days to help heal leaky gut and cure autoimmune disease.

Raw Cultured Dairy: contains both probiotics and short-chain fatty acids that can help heal the gut. Pastured Kefir, yogurt, Amasai (Amasai is a cultured milk beverage with the consistency of liquid yogurt; it provides high-quality proteins, vitamins, minerals, enzymes, probiotics and healthy fats), butter, and raw cheese are some of the best.

Fermented Vegetables: contain organic acids that balance intestinal pH and probiotics to support the gut. Sauerkraut, kimchi, and kvass are excellent sources.

Coconut Products: all Coconut products are especially good for your gut. The medium-chain fatty acids in coconut are easier to digest than those in other fats so they work well for leaky gut. Also, coconut kefir contains probiotics that support your digestive system.

Sprouted Seeds: chia seeds, flaxseeds, and hemp seeds that have been sprouted are great sources of fiber that can help support the growth of beneficial bacteria. But if you have severe leaky gut, you may need to start out getting your fiber from steamed vegetables and fruit.

Consuming foods that have omega-3 fats are also beneficial and anti-inflammatory foods like grass-fed beef, lamb, and wild-caught fish like salmon or mackerel.

I had the good fortune to participate in the Healthy Gut Summit this year and learned some great information from a variety of experts in the field on nutrition and natural medicine. The host for the summit was Dr. Josh Axe, a certified doctor of natural medicine and clinical nutritionist with a passion to help people get healthy by using food as medicine.

Dr. Axe, along with Sayer Ji, founder of GreenMedInfo.com and a researcher on natural health and gut health, recommended several supplements and herbal remedies that can also affect the health your leaky gut.

Step 3: Add supplements and herbs.

Probiotics are the most important supplement to take because it helps replenish good bacteria and moves out bad bacteria. Probiotics in both food and supplement form are most effective. I see people in my practice who only follow part of the protocol in healing their leaky gut syndrome by removing the damaging irritants or trigger foods. The part they often leave out is feeding their gut with beneficial bacteria that will keep bad bacteria at bay. My recommendation is to load up on both probiotic-rich foods and take at least fifty billion units of probiotics daily from a high-quality brand. One that I use is a probiotic/prebiotic and digestive enzyme combined.

Digestive enzymes (one or two capsules at the beginning of each meal) ensure that foods are fully digested, decreasing the chance that partially digested foods particles and proteins are damaging your gut wall. As mentioned previously, if you can find enzymes combined with your probiotic it makes it that easier to take on a daily basis.

L-Glutamine is critical for any program designed to heal leaky gut. Glutamine powder is an essential amino acid supplement that is anti-inflammatory and necessary for the growth and repair of your intestinal lining. L-glutamine benefits include coating your cell walls and acting as a repellent to irritants. Take two to five grams twice daily.

Licorice root (DGL) is an adaptogenic herb that helps balance cortisol levels and improves acid production in the stomach. DGL supports the body's natural processes for maintaining the mucosal lining of the stomach and duodenum. This herb is especially beneficial if someone's leaky gut is being caused by emotional stress. Recommended dose is five hundred milligrams twice daily.

Quercetin works by sealing the gut because it supports creation of tight junction proteins. It also stabilizes mast cells and reduces the release of histamine, which is common in food intolerance. New studies have also shown its effectiveness in healing ulcerative colitis. The recommended dose is five hundred milligrams three times daily with meals.

Peppermint oil capsules have been long used to reduce stomachaches, soothe digestive issues, and clear respiratory tracts, and it as antimicrobial properties. To relieve IBS and for temporary use, it is suggested to use two to three capsules a day between meals and is not recommended for daily, casual use.

Jerusalem artichokes contain inulin, a type of prebiotic fiber that has been credited with a number of health benefits due to its medicinal properties. Many of these health benefits can be attributed to the ability of inulin to stimulate the growth of bifidobacteria. Naturally present in the large intestine, bifidobacteria fight harmful bacteria in the intestines, prevent constipation, gives the immune system a boost and helps reduce intestinal concentrations of certain carcinogenic enzymes. "Jerusalem Artichokes: Health Benefits & Nutritional Properties." *Health Benefits & Nutritional Properties of Jerusalem Artichokes*. Amazon Services LLC Associate Program, n.d. Web. 28 Jan. 2016. <http://www.healwithfood.org/health-benefits/jerusalem-artichokes.php>.

Turmeric is anti-inflammatory to the mucous membranes, which coat the throat, lungs, stomach, and intestines. It decreases congestion and inflammation from stagnant mucous membranes. People with the following conditions could benefit from regular use of turmeric: IBS, colitis, Crohn's disease, diarrhea, and post-Giardia or postsalmonella conditions. It can also reduce the itching and inflammation that accompany hemorrhoids and anal fissures. This herb would be useful to follow up antibiotic treatments, in addition to acidophilus and garlic as it helps to improve the intestinal flora and acts as an antibacterial.

Be sure to consult your physician before taking any supplements to avoid any possible reaction with any medication or protocol you may currently be on. If you can follow this protocol, you will be well on your way to successfully healing your gut health for the long term.

Step 4: Change your lifestyle.

In addition to all of the foods you should eliminate or add in and the supplements and probiotics that will strengthen your gut, making changes in your daily lifestyle is also important.

Reduce Chronic Stress: "The connection between the gut and our psychology is deep and is kind of like a two-way street. On one side of the street, gastrointestinal inflammation and infection can contribute to things like depression and brain fog. On the other, mental stress or trauma can cause intestinal permeability or leaky gut," according to Donna Gates, MEd, ABAAHP.

Psychological stress can do more than influence the integrity of our own cells. Scientific studies have found that the bacteria living inside of us can actually detect whether we actually feel stress. When we experience mental, emotional, or physical stress, we release stress hormones like cortisol and norepinephrine. These stress hormones are meant to protect us during potentially dangerous events (fight or flight). They move energy stores into the muscle, increasing our heart rate and our breathing. In the process, cortisol and norepinephrine shut down our digestive and immune systems.

If you have chronic stress in your daily life, it is important to identify the sources of that stress and then find ways to reduce it—permanently. A great way to identify the sources of your stress and to work through them is with a certified health coach. Health coaches are trained to help you identify and manage your nutritional needs, and they will coach you through areas of your life that may be inhibiting your path to sustainable, long-term health.

Schedule downtime: This may need to be addressed with the same people who suffer from chronic stress. Very often this person has a classic "type A" personality who may be a bit of a workaholic or someone who is overcommitted and does not make time to take time off. Scheduling downtime is imperative to give your body and mind a break! You cannot fill someone else's cup when yours is empty.

Once your trigger foods are eliminated, healing foods are reintroduced, and your lifestyle changes include a major reduction in stress, you will be well on your way to a healthy gut and a reduction in the symptoms of any autoimmune diseases that may be affecting you.

So after you cleaned out your cabinets and pantry and gotten rid of all things with gluten or any other allergens in them, your kitchen may look pretty bare. Now you must head to the grocery store and restock with healthy food items that will no longer make you sick. This may feel like a daunting challenge at first. Do not worry, though. I will walk you through an easy way to manage the grocery store and stock your home with good food.

Here are few tips on what to do before you even head out to the store. It will make life a bit easier to have a game plan, and you will focus on what you need to buy for the week before you hit the store.

Know Your Local Grocers
Do a little bit of research and find how which ones carry the best selection of organic foods, gluten-free foods, and so on. Not all neighborhoods have a Whole Foods or a Trader Joe's, so call the store and ask if it carries these products.

Look for Online Retailers to Fill in the Blanks
If you cannot find certain products at your local grocery store, find online retailers that do offer a variety of gluten-free or allergy-free products. One of my favorites is called Thrive Market. Their site allows you to choose the allergies or preferences for your family and then will offer selections of products in all categories that are free from those items you may be allergic to. It is a subscription-based group, and once you pay the initial fee, it ships products directly to your front door. Very convenient! There are many others, so do some research to see which ones offer more of the products you are looking for and at the price point that works with your budget.

Shop Your Local Farmers' Markets
Because the idea is to eat clean and to incorporate as many organic fruits and vegetables, as well as organic and locally grown meats, into your diet, the farmers' market is a great option. You can find anything from fruits and veggies to fresh eggs, local honey, grass-fed beef, and much, much more. It is also a great way to support your local community. Depending on what part of the country you live in, you may have access to farmers' markets just a few months of the year or year-round. In any case, take advantage of the offerings as much as possible.

Plan in Advance
It is easy to head to the store and just start buying everything you think you may need for the week, but it really is best if you have a plan in advance. I highly suggest, particularly if you are dealing with a new diagnosis, that you think out what meals you want to prepare for the week and purchase the items accordingly. If you are planning to buy organic as well, going to the store weekly works best because organic fruits and veggies do not keep nearly as long as those with preservatives. You don't want to spend good money on beautiful organic products just to have them go bad after a week.

Start out with some recipes that fit your new dietary needs and plan them out for the week. Are there some recipes that you can prepare that will allow you some leftovers? Those are great to repurpose for lunch the next day or for dinner again. There are some great websites available as well that offer really easy recipes for busy families that have gluten-free slow cooker freezer ideas. You can prepare several meals in advance, stick them in the freezer, and then pull them out for an easy-to-prepare meal during the week. These type of meals are easy to shop for, and you can buy all the ingredients at once, prepare the meals, and then forget about it until you are ready to eat!

The good news is that all grocery stores carry a large number of products that are naturally gluten-free—foods like fruits, vegetables, meat, fresh poultry, fish, nuts and seeds, beans, rice, potatoes, cheese, and milk. There are more items than that, but you get the picture.

Today, because the focus on gluten-free, dairy-free, and allergen-free foods is greater, many stores now have dedicated sections that feature these products. For example, I live in Texas, and we have several grocers here that have dedicated gluten-free sections as well as all natural and organic food sections! One local Kroger store has such an enormous offering of frozen gluten-free products that it takes up an entire wall in the store, which is very impressive!

Sometimes gluten-free products are mixed in with their regular counterparts. As an example, one of my local stores mixes gluten-free pasta in with regular pasta in the aisle as well as in the dedicated gluten-free section, but it is nice to know that I can find it in both places. The best thing to do is ask the store manager where those products are shelved so you can find them easily and get to know where to find them in your favorite store.

One of the things I love about Trader Joe's is that it actually will provide you with a printed list of all of its gluten-free items. Talk about being customer-friendly and making it easy to shop its stores. Those kind of resources will make your shopping experience easier and more convenient until you get to know what you are looking for and where to find it.

How to Shop the Grocery Store

A good rule of thumb is to shop the perimeter of the grocery store. This is a good general strategy to help you buy healthy foods and avoid the "junk" that is often found in the center of the store. Most grocery stores are laid out pretty much the same. Some may flip the layout from one side to the other, but the structure of the store is pretty standard.

Your **first stop should be the produce section.** Be sure to look for the colors of the rainbow. The more colorful your fruits and veggies are, the more health benefits you will find from them. Look for the dark green, deep orange, red, and purple fruits and veggies. Not only will you get more nutrients from these foods, but they also look beautiful on your plate. The more color, the better! When you can find organics, consider buying them as well, and don't forget to wash all fruits and vegetables well once you get home and before you put them in the fridge or before you store them.

Somewhere after the produce section, you will likely **pass through the bakery section of the store and just keep on going!** Nine times out of ten you will not find gluten-free items in the bakery, so it is better to avoid it altogether. You will find gluten-free bread and baked goods elsewhere in the store, and I will tell you where to keep an eye out for those.

Next up is usually the section where you find **meat, fish, and poultry.** This is your next stop. Fresh meat, poultry, and fish are great sources of protein, minerals, and even a place to find good fats, such as those you will find in wild salmon and mackerel. Be sure to leave behind any of the prepackaged meals that have been marinated, coated, or battered. These may all contain gluten and hidden forms of gluten. You can also look at the deli counter for fresh plain meats and cheeses.

However, you should avoid any mixed salads or composite meats because they may also contain hidden forms of gluten along with a variety of preservatives and other "junk" ingredients. Keep in mind that some processed lunchmeats contain gluten to be sure to ask the deli manager or read the labels. Also ask if a slicer is dedicated to gluten-free products. If one is not, ask if the clerk can use a knife to cut off a block of the meat for you in the weight you are looking for, and then you can slice the meat at home yourself to avoid the risk of any cross-contamination from the deli slicer.

Next up on your trip around the store is likely to be the **dairy section.** This is generally a safe zone, unless of course you are either lactose intolerant or if you have a dairy allergy. The good news is that many stores now offer options like almond milk, soy milk, and cashew milk along with their regular and lactose-free options. The same goes for yogurt and cheese, so be sure to ask the store manager where any dairy-free options are. Sometimes they will be mixed in with the dairy options and sometimes will have a separate area within the refrigerated section. For those of you who have gluten issues, be sure to read packaging here too as some cheese sauces or flavored cream cheeses may have fillers that contain gluten or flavoring agents with the same gluten risk.

The refrigerated section of the grocery store may also be where you will find a dedicated area for gluten-free items such as cookie dough, piecrust, and pizza crust. These items may sometimes be in the frozen section, so double-check with the store manager to find out where these products are in your store.

Bulk bins in the store may seem like a good area for gluten-free options. However, you will want to consider cross-contamination here because other customers may have innocently used a scoop from a gluten-containing bin into one with gluten-free product, and then you are at risk. **It is best to avoid the bulk bins** altogether and to purchase the prepackaged version of these items from other parts of the store.

Speaking of which, let's look at the **packaged goods section** of the store. This area makes up a large section of the store, and most likely, you will need products from there. My caution is to read the labels on everything! Here you will find rice, beans, breakfast cereals, and baking needs. Be sure to look for those items that are gluten-free. This is also where you will find the gluten-free products section so just be aware of what is on the label and make smart choices. Plain versions of dried herbs and spices are best and avoid those prepackaged spice blends as they may contain gluten. Sauce packets for salad dressing, seasoning for taco meat, and so on are all likely to contain gluten. Some are gluten-free, so look closely for those options.

The **frozen section** is another big part of most grocery stores. Frozen fruits and veggies are usually OK as long as they do not contain sauces. Also, look for plain frozen meat, poultry, and fish and avoid anything that is breaded or battered unless it is specifically labeled gluten-free. You may also find here frozen gluten-free breads, muffins, waffles, microwaveable meals, and gluten-free pizza. For those with dairy issues, if you were an ice cream person, see if you can find some of the great soy- or coconut-based frozen treats. They are delicious and are a great way to satisfy your sweet tooth. Again, read all labels carefully here.

Two other areas of the store where you will want to use caution are the **personal-care** and **medication aisles** and the **alcohol section.** It may not seem like it would be necessary, but many products contain gluten. You may find it in everything from body lotion to shampoo, lipstick to vitamins. Ask your doctor if a list of potential products that may contain gluten is available and, once again, read every label. There are personal-care product lines available that do not contain gluten or many other allergens. Companies, like Arbonne, are great resources online because they offer products from nutritionals to skin care, from supplements to cosmetics that are all gluten-free, dairy-free, soy-free, non-GMO, and they also never test on animals. Research is very helpful in this area to see what other companies are making these kinds of products so you can convert your entire household, not just your kitchen and pantry.

Alcohol is another area to pay special attention to. You will want to avoid any alcohol that is made from wheat, barley, or rye. There are now many gluten-free options available from craft beer to vodka so again, do your research and read the labels.

Is Gluten-Free Shopping More Expensive?

In one word, yes. It can be more expensive to shop gluten-free as the cost to produce gluten-free products is sometimes costlier. Sometimes manufacturers have to charge more because it takes more to use gluten-free grains and to process them in special ways and with separate equipment.

Here are some tips on how to do cut costs at the grocery store:

Never go to the store hungry: You will buy less and make better choices.

Plan meals in advance: Buy only what you need for the week.

Buy seasonal foods: Buy foods in season, and they will be fresher and cheaper.
Make food from scratch: Premade foods are typically more expensive than cooking from scratch is. Baked goods, in particular, can be pricey in the store, so it is great to make them at home from scratch.

Buy in bulk: Once you figure out which products you like best, check online or in warehouse stores to see what you can buy in bulk. Things like meats, poultry and fruits and veggies are also good in bulk. You can store them in freezer safe containers and keep in the freezer for several weeks.

Use coupons and special offers: Get on some mailing lists for gluten-free or specialty retailers and take advantage of their coupons and flyers online or in store. Trader Joe's and Whole Foods also offer coupons and special circulars so keep track of any discounts available there.

Apply for a tax deduction: Did you know that you can apply for a tax deduction for the special gluten-free products you buy? There is now a special tax deduction available if you have to follow a gluten-free diet for medical reasons! You will need to submit an official written diagnosis from your doctor along with your tax records or give it to your accountant for them to submit.

You will need to keep all of your receipts so you can compare the cost of the gluten-free product versus the regular version of the product. This can be very time-consuming, but it will certainly help with costs at the end of the year.

Another way to cut cost on gluten-free foods is to learn to **create menu plans and meals that do not have to include expensive gluten-free foods like pasta or bread.** Eating whole, fresh foods like lean protein, meat, poultry, fish, and fresh fruits and veggies can help you avoid the need to buy a lot of other costly products that are also full of carbohydrates and sugars. Eating clean is a good way to go in general because it will be healthier and less expensive.

Talk to your dietician, nutritionist or health coach to help you prepare smart meal plans that will suit the needs of you and your family without being a detriment to your family budget.

Chapter 11: Favorite Gluten-Free and Dairy-Free Recipes and How to Play "Kitchen Improv"

Lemon Garlic Shrimp. Butternut Squash Lasagna. Sunday Morning Breakfast Quiche. Sweet Corn and Zucchini Pie. Kale Salad with Chicken. Glazed Brussels Sprouts. Crockpot Balsamic Chicken. Spaghetti Pie. Hummingbird Cake.

These are some of my very favorite recipes that I have made for years and have had to adapt to accommodate either gluten-free eating or a gluten-free and dairy-free lifestyle. After I was diagnosed with celiac and was subsequently diagnosed with the dairy allergy, I wanted to learn how to continue making my favorite dishes but substituting new ingredients to compensate for those I was no longer able to eat.

Sometimes it is easier to begin with meals that are naturally gluten-free. Try grilling a protein (meat, poultry, or fish) with some easy, gluten-free seasonings. Make a beautiful salad or steam some vegetables to go along with it. If you want some starch with your meal, try a baked potato or some steamed brown rice. Pretty simple.

Once you are comfortable with recipes like that, try something a bit harder and make some simple substitutions. For example, if you love pasta, when you do your shopping, buy some gluten-free pasta and a gluten-free pasta sauce. Again, pretty simple to put together and be sure to look at the cooking directions on the pasta because it cooks longer than most other pastas. If you love meatloaf, try the same recipe you always use and substitute gluten-free breadcrumbs for regular ones. You and your family likely won't even know the difference.

The next step is to really experiment in the kitchen with things like making gluten-free pancakes or gluten-free bread or making batter for fish or chicken from gluten-free flour.

The same principle applies to any allergy that you may learning to manage. For example, I also have a dairy allergy, so instead of using regular milk, I will use either soy, almond, cashew, or coconut milk based on the recipe and what kind of flavor or consistency I am trying to achieve. I use vegan cheese instead of regular cheese for numerous recipes. I like the product Go Veggie, which has sliced singles as well as shredded vegan "cheese." The product tastes good and actually melts like real cheese. One of my favorite treats is a gluten-free/dairy-free grilled cheese sandwich and a bowl of homemade tomato soup! If you have kids with gluten and/or dairy allergies, this will be a great go-to meal for you, and they will love it.

Don't fear that you will need fancy kitchen tools and appliances to make gluten-free cooking easy. All you need is an open mind and a positive attitude to get started. Some recipes may turn out really well the first time, and some may not. The key is not to get discouraged but keep practicing with recipes and ingredients until you get it right.

One of the first things I tried was the "Basic Gluten Free Flour Mix" from the book *Guide to Gluten Free Eating* from the Mayo Clinic. This recipe can be used as a substitute for regular wheat flour. The consistency is OK, but there are so many one-to-one gluten-free flours available that taste great without having to mix them yourself. My personal favorite brand is Pamela's gluten-free flour. It works so well in pancakes, cookies, breads, gravy, and in batters for frying. You can order it online from a variety of sources, and the pricing is reasonable as well.

Over the next few pages, you will find some of my favorite recipes that have substitutions in them, either gluten or gluten and dairy. I hope you will experiment with them, try some of your own favorites with substitutions, and improvise in the kitchen!

Kale Salad with Chicken (gluten-free and dairy-free)

- 1 large bunch of kale
- Juice from 1/2 orange
- 2 tablespoons extra virgin olive oil
- 1 cup walnuts
- 1/2 cup dried cranberries, unsweetened
- 1 large chicken breast
- 1 clove garlic, minced

Wash, dry, and chop the kale. Drizzle orange juice and 1 tablespoon olive oil to coat the leaves. Massage into the kale. Add walnuts and cranberries and let sit for at least 30 minutes. Heat 1 teaspoon olive oil in the sauté pan over medium heat. Add garlic, and when garlic is slightly browned, add the chicken. Cook about 5 minutes; then flip and cook another 5 minutes to cook through fully. In another a sauté pan use 1 teaspoon olive oil and sauté the kale, cranberries, and walnuts until the kale becomes a bit wilted (but not overly so). Serve warm.

Lemon Garlic Shrimp and Vegetables (gluten-free and dairy-free)

- 4 teaspoons extra virgin olive oil, divided
- 2 large red bell peppers, diced
- 2 pounds asparagus, trimmed and cut into 1-inch lengths
- 2 teaspoons freshly grated lemon zest
- 1/2 teaspoon salt, divided
- 5 cloves garlic, minced
- 1 pound raw shrimp (26–30 count shrimp), peeled and deveined
- 1 cup gluten-free reduced-sodium chicken broth
- 1 teaspoon cornstarch
- 2 tablespoons lemon juice
- 2 tablespoons chopped fresh parsley

Heat 2 teaspoons oil in a large nonstick skillet over medium-high heat. Add bell peppers, asparagus, lemon zest, and 1/4 teaspoon salt and cook, stirring occasionally, until just beginning to soften, about 6 minutes. Transfer the vegetables to a bowl; cover to keep warm.

Add the remaining 2 teaspoons oil and garlic to the pan and cook, stirring, until fragrant, about 30 seconds. Add shrimp and cook, stirring, for 1 minute. Whisk broth and cornstarch in a small bowl until smooth and add to the pan along with the remaining 1/4 teaspoon salt. Cook, stirring, until the sauce has thickened slightly and the shrimp are pink and just cooked through, about 2 minutes more. Remove from the heat. Stir in lemon juice and parsley. Serve the shrimp and sauce over the vegetables.

Butternut Squash and Kale Lasagna (gluten-free)

- 1/4 cup water
- 1 package (12 ounces) pre-chopped fresh butternut squash
- 3 cups pre-chopped kale
- 1 tablespoon olive oil
- 1 1/2 tablespoons minced garlic
- 1/4 cup all-purpose gluten-free flour—Pamela's is best
- 3/4 cups 1 percent low-fat milk, divided (I substituted cashew milk here, but soy or coconut milk will do also)
- 4 ounces gruyere cheese, shredded and divided
- 1 ounce Parmigiano-Reggiano cheese, grated
- 1/2 teaspoon salt
- 1/4 teaspoon black pepper
- Cooking spray
- 6 no-boil gluten-free lasagna noodles
- 4 tablespoons chopped pecans

Preheat oven to 450°F. Combine 1/4 cup water and squash in an eight-inch square glass or ceramic baking dish. Cover tightly with plastic wrap; pierce plastic wrap two to three times. Microwave on high for 5 minutes or until tender; drain. Combine squash and kale in a large bowl. Wipe dish dry.

Heat a medium saucepan over medium heat. Add oil to pan; swirl to coat. Add garlic; cook 2 minutes or until garlic begins to brown, stirring occasionally. Weigh or lightly spoon flour into a dry measuring cup; level with a knife. Combine flour and 1/2 cup milk in a small bowl, stirring with a whisk until smooth. Add milk mixture and remaining two 1/4 cups milk to pan; increase heat to medium-high. Bring to a boil; cook 1 minute or until thickened, stirring frequently. Remove from heat. Stir in 1 ounce gruyere, Parmigiano-Reggiano cheese, salt, and pepper; stir until cheese melts.

Coat baking dish with cooking spray. Spread 1/3 cup milk mixture in bottom of dish. Arrange 2 noodles over milk mixture; top with half of squash mixture and 2/3 cup milk mixture. Repeat layers once, ending with remaining noodles and remaining milk mixture. Cover with foil; bake at 450° for 15 minutes. Remove foil; sprinkle remaining Gruyere and pecans over top. Bake, uncovered, at 450° for 10 minutes or until lightly browned and sauce is bubbly. Let stand 5 minutes then serve.

Sunday Morning Breakfast Quiches
(gluten-free and dairy-free)

- 10 eggs
- 1 cup coconut milk
- 1/2 cup of finely chopped broccoli
- 1/2 cup of chopped mushrooms
- 8 slices of cooked bacon, chopped
- 1 cup of Go Veggie shredded cheese (vegan cheese)
- Coconut oil
- Muffin pan or glass baking dish

Preheat the oven to 350°F. Whisk eggs and incorporate the coconut milk (shake can well before pouring) into the eggs. Lightly grease each muffin cup with coconut oil. Distribute the bacon and veggies evenly into each muffin cup. Fill each cup with the egg mixture to a uniform fill. Bake at 350 degrees for about 30 minutes (depends on your oven). Check to make sure eggs have set firmly before removing from oven. They made need another 5 to 10 minutes depending on your oven temperature distribution. Allow to cool for about 5 minutes before removing from the muffin pan and serve.

You can use any veggies/meats combo you want to with this recipe. You can also add in some regular cheese to the egg mixture if you prefer. I use the vegan cheese to make this gluten-free and dairy-free. These can be stored in a Ziploc or airtight container for up to five days, and they reheat beautifully. I have done them for brunch in large muffin tins that have design in the bottom and serve on top of a nicely dressed mixed green salad for a lovely brunch dish or you can also just pour the egg mixture into a glass baking dish and then cut into squares for serving.

Vegetable Bake

- 4 tablespoons butter
- 1 yellow onion, diced
- 2 ears sweet corn
- 2 large yellow or green zucchini, diced (about 4 cups)
- 8 ounces sliced mushrooms
- 1 tablespoon dried basil
- 1 teaspoon dried oregano
- 1/2 teaspoon salt
- 12 ounces Daiya dairy free shredded cheese
- 4 eggs, beaten

Preheat the oven to 375°F. Heat the butter in a large, deep skillet over medium-high heat. Add the onions, zucchini, and mushrooms. While the veggies sauté, cut the corn kernels off the cob. Add them to the pan and continue to sauté until the veggies are soft, 5 to 10 minutes. Remove from heat.

Add the basil, oregano, and salt. Stir once to combine. In a separate bowl, mix the cheese and the beaten egg. Line a pie pan (nine inches or larger) with parchment paper or grease a pan with nonstick spray. Transfer the sautéed veggies into the dish and then cover with the cheese/egg mixture. Using a fork, turn the cheese/egg mixture into the veggies to incorporate. Arrange the top so the sliced zucchini slices lay flat and look nice. Top with a little extra cheese for looks, cover with greased foil, and bake for 20 minutes. Remove foil and bake for an additional 5 minutes to brown the top. Let stand for 10 to 15 minutes before cutting into slices.

The pie will bubble up a little bit as it bakes, so put a pan under to catch drips if it's really full. Also, there was a little extra watery-ness (about 2 tablespoons) in the bottom of my pan when I sliced it, but the pieces held together perfectly…so no big deal. I think the moisture could be prevented by just being a little more patient before cutting. Sprinkle with chopped parsley and/or basil for a nice fresh finish if you like. ENJOY!

Crockpot Balsamic Chicken

- 1 teaspoon garlic powder
- 1 teaspoon dried basil
- 1/2 teaspoon pepper
- 2 teaspoons dried minced onion
- 4 garlic cloves, minced
- 1 tablespoon extra virgin olive oil
- 1/2 cup gluten-free balsamic vinegar
- 8 boneless, skinless chicken thighs or breasts
- Sprinkle of fresh chopped parsley

Combine the first four dry spices in a small bowl and spread over chicken on both sides. Set aside. Pour olive oil and garlic on the bottom of the slow cooker. Place chicken on top. Pour balsamic vinegar over the chicken. Cover and cook on high for 4 hours. Sprinkle the fresh parsley on top to serve.

Glazed Brussels Sprouts

- 1 pound of fresh Brussels sprouts (cut in half, lengthwise)
- 1 1/2 cups of low-sodium vegetable or chicken stock
- 1/8 cup of gluten-free balsamic glaze (Fini is my favorite)
- 1/2 cup of dried cranberries
- 1/2 cup of sliced almonds
- 3 tablespoons of olive oil

Wash the sprouts and allow them to dry before you prepare the dish. You do not want to extra moisture in the sprouts. Sauté the sprouts over medium-high heat in the olive oil until the start to get golden brown. Add in 1 cup of stock and turn heat down to simmer. Cover the sprouts and let them steam until they become soft, approximately 15 minutes, stirring occasionally.

Add in the dried cranberries and allow them to plump up, approximately 10 minutes. Drizzle the balsamic glaze over the sprouts and stir until they are coated. Let cook until the sprouts get caramelized and start to crisp up. When you are ready to serve, sprinkle on the almonds, and you are all set to enjoy!

Hummingbird Cake
(Light and gluten-free)

- Vegetable cooking spray
- 3 cups plus 2 teaspoons gluten-free (one-to-one) flour, divided
- 1 teaspoon baking soda
- 1/2 teaspoon salt
- 1 3/4 cups sugar
- 1 teaspoon ground cinnamon
- 2 large eggs
- 1/2 cup unsweetened applesauce
- 3 tablespoons vegetable oil
- 1 3/4 cups mashed banana (about 5 or 6 bananas)
- 1 1/2 teaspoons vanilla extract
- 1 can (8 ounces) crushed pineapple, un-drained
- Light cream-cheese frosting
- 1 cup of walnuts (finely chopped)

Coat three round nine-inch cake pans with cooking spray; sprinkle 2 teaspoons gluten-free flour evenly into pans, shaking to coat.

Combine remaining 3 cups gluten-free flour and next four ingredients in a large bowl. Stir together eggs, applesauce, and oil; add to flour mixture, stirring just until dry ingredients are moistened. (Do not beat.) Stir in mashed banana, vanilla extract, crushed pineapple with the juice and 3/4 cup of the walnuts.

Pour batter evenly into prepared pans. Bake at 350°F for 23 to 25 minutes or until a wooden pick inserted in center comes out clean. Cool layers in pans on wire racks for 10 minutes. Remove layers from pans; cool completely on wire racks.

Spread light cream-cheese frosting between layers and on top, leaving sides of the cake free of frosting, and sprinkle remaining walnuts on the top of the cake. If you want to add the extra calories, go ahead and frost the sides of the cake as well.

Conclusion

If your new diagnosis—whether it be a new food allergy or medical condition—has you down, know that there are many ways to find support and many other people who are empathetic to your situation. The most important thing I have learned over the years is that you can overcome anything with the right attitude, the ability to do research, and the love and support of family and friends.

It is normal to feel anxious, nervous, or even scared with a new diagnosis. Don't beat yourself up for feeling that way. Take one day at a time, and it will not seem quite so daunting.

Feelings of fatigue, being overwhelmed, chronic sadness, insomnia, anxiety, depression, and even headaches can be very common in people with celiac disease. Studies have shown the tie between our brain, our gut, and (as referenced in chapter 9 gut health is imperative, so when we have issues that affect our digestive tract, they can also pose psychological issues.

Once gluten is fully removed from your diet, you will begin to see those feelings of sadness, anxiety, and depression subside. Here are some final tips on what you can do to create a full and happy life for yourself and your family.

Take Care of Yourself

Be sure to follow your new dietary lifestyle and be diligent about it. The health benefits will far outweigh the frustration and challenges at the beginning. I always say that I never realized how badly I felt until I did not feel that way anymore. Get plenty of exercise, get plenty of sleep, and drink a lot of water. Overall physical health will always help to improve your mental health.

Avoid Negativity

Getting caught up in one's own head and focusing on the negative aspects of a new diagnosis rather than the positive ones is easy. Instead, remind yourself that eating gluten-free and dairy-free is better for sustainable good health in the long term. By following the correct diet, you remove congestion, inflammation, and harm from your body, and that is a great thing. Cultivate relationships with others in your situation, and find support groups in your neighborhood and online. There are some negative people in those group as well, so be sure to avoid them, and spend time with those who are supportive and uplifting.

Talk It Out

When you have feelings of frustration, or if you are struggling, find someone to talk to who will understand your situation. Health coaches are great resources because they are there to listen to you and to let you talk about what your needs are. They are trained in a wide variety of areas and can really help you to create an environment where you can voice your concerns, share your triumphs, and find new information to continue building on your own health success.

Be Prepared

This is the most important tip for me as I have learned to be prepared for whatever situation I may find myself in: Be prepared for your weekly meals. Be prepared for your trip to the grocery store. Be prepared for business and personal travel, and be prepared to know what to look and ask for when walking into a situation where you are not sure of what may be served. I always carry a "survival kit" with me as well.

My survival kit includes homemade trail mix or other gluten-free snacks, protein shake packs, an extra large travel tissue pack in case of a bathroom emergency, and medication to treat diarrhea or constipation.

Educate Others

You are now going to be the expert on your condition (or that of a family member), so be sure to educate the rest of your family and your friends. Most will want to be helpful and supportive, but they may not know how to be. Share with them what you can and cannot eat, and let them know it is OK to ask you more questions.

Enjoy Your Life

Living with celiac, food allergies, or any dietary restriction will pose its share of challenges. The key is to be patient with yourself and others, to have a positive outlook, and to know that learning to manage anything new is a process. Enjoy your health, and enjoy your life.

About the Author

Heidi L. Smith, CCWS, CINHC, CMP, is a certified corporate wellness specialist, certified integrative nutrition health coach, a certified meeting professional, and the founder and chief-executive officer of the Integrative Wellness Studio in Greater Houston area.

Heidi spent more than twenty-five years in the meetings industry and was a classic "road warrior" for many of those years, traveling around the country for her job. After being diagnosed with celiac disease and other food allergies, she found it hard to manage being on the road and to stick to a dietary lifestyle that had so many restrictions in it.

After talking with other colleagues who were experiencing issues with various food allergies and digestive issues, she has helped numerous people find that they too had celiac disease or gluten sensitivities that had gone undetected for years. Finding joy in being able to help others to get well sparked her interest in learning more about autoimmune disease and food allergies and about how to manage the consequential dietary needs.

In order to help others more fully, she decided to make a major life change and quit the meetings industry to pursue a training program with the Institute for Integrative Nutrition in New York. She received her certification as an Integrative Nutrition Health Coach and opened her practice, the Integrative Wellness Studio in Chicago and eventually in Houston.

The Integrative Wellness Studio offers one-on-one health coaching programs to assist people in finding sustainable health through lifestyle and nutrition. Heidi leads classes and workshops on a variety of topics, develops wellness programs, and speaks to groups about nutrition and developing a healthier lifestyle.

Heidi lives in Houston, Texas, with her husband, Dennis, and two dogs, Wally and Agador. Her stepson, Austin, is finishing his engineering degree in Louisiana, and because Heidi and Dennis are empty nesters, they enjoy cooking, golfing, playing tennis, and traveling. Heidi is also involved in the community doing volunteer work with a number of charities, including her favorite work helping to rescue stray animals in the local neighborhood.

Resources

Axe, J. *"4 Steps to Heal Leaky Gut and Autoimmune Disease"*. Draxe.com. Accessed January 5, 2016. http://www.draxe.com.

Gates, D. *"Healing Leaky Gut: Prevent Chronic Inflammation."* Body Ecology.com. Accessed February 2, 2016. http://www.bodyecology.com/articles/healing-leaky-gut.

Dumke, N. *The Ultimate Food Allergy Cookbook & Survival Guide: How to Cook with Ease for a Food Allergy Diet and Recover Good Health.* Louisville, CO: Adapt Books, 2006.

Edwards, M. *"Gluten, Candida, Leaky Gut Syndrome and Autoimmune Diseases."* Organiclifestyle.com. Last Modified April 20, 2015. http://www.organiclifestyle.com.

"Eosinophilic Esophagitis Diets. Six Food Elimination Diet." Accessed February 2, 2016. http://www.eosinophilicesophagitis.org.

Fitterman, L. *"When Dairy Intolerance Joins Celiac Disease."* Last modified 2012. http://www.allergicliving.com.

Kaslow, J. *"Leaky Gut Syndrome."* Last modified 2016. http://drkaslow.com.

Murray, J., MD, and J. See, LD, eds. Mayo Clinic. *Guide to Eating Gluten Free.* New York, NY: Time Home Entertainment, 2014.

Rosenthal, J. *Integrative Nutrition: Feed Your Hunger for Health & Happiness.* Austin, TX: Greenleaf Book Group, LLC, 2014.

"Jerusalem Artichokes: Health Benefits & Nutritional Properties." *Health Benefits & Nutritional Properties of Jerusalem Artichokes.* Amazon Services LLC Associate Program, n.d. Web. 28 Jan. 2016. <http://www.healwithfood.org/health-benefits/jerusalem-artichokes.php>.

"About Anaphylaxis." Foodallergy.org. Accessed January 15, 2016. http://www.foodallergy.org/anaphylaxis.

Fitterman, L. *"When Dairy Intolerance Joins Celiac Disease."* Allergicliving.com. Fall 2012. http://wwwallergicliving.com

"Eosinophilic Esophagitis (EE) or (EOE)." AAAAI.org. Accessed January 15, 2016. http://www.aaaai.org/conditions-and-treatments/library/allergy-library/eosinophilic-esophagitis.aspx

"Candida." Merriam-Webster.com. Merriam-Webster, n.d. Web. 9 Mar. 2016.

Weil, Andrew, M.D. *"What is Leaky Gut?"* drweil.com. Last modified December, 12, 2005. http://www.Drweil.com/drw/u/QAA361058/what-is-leaky-gut

www.ingramcontent.com/pod-product-compliance
Lightning Source LLC
Chambersburg PA
CBHW071247280526
45788CB00004B/1620